Homemade Beauty Products

Over 50 All Natural Homemade Recipes For Face Masks, Facial Cleansers & Face Creams

All contents copyrighted © 2014 of Lorraine White. All rights reserved worldwide. No part of this publication may be reproduced in any form or by any means, including scanning, photocopying, or otherwise without prior written permission of the copyright holder.

In no event shall the author be liable for any direct, indirect, incidental, punitive or consequential damages of any kind whatsoever with respect to the service, the materials and the products contained within. This book is not a substitute for professional medical or skin care advice.

Table of Contents

	Page
Introduction	1
Everyday Products Full of Harmful Chemicals	2
Making Your Own Beauty Products	4
How To Be Beautiful – Top Tips	5
Basic Set Up & Equipment Needed	8
Homemade Facial Cleansers – Intro	9
Super Simple Cleanser	10
Moisturizing Face Cleanser	11
Skin Restoring Fruit Cleanser	12
Skin Smoothing Flour Cleanser	13
Tea Tree Cleanser	14
Lavender Anti-Aging Face Cleanser	15
Fresh Orange Cleanser	16
Acne Helping Cleanser	17
Simple Strawberry Cleanser	18
Aloe Gel Face Wash	19
Baking Soda Cleanser	20
Yogurt Face Cleanser	21
Avocado Dry Skin Cleanser	22
Cucumber Face Cleanser	23
Lemon & Honey Cleanser	24
Homemade Face Masks – Intro	25
Almond & Honey Face Mask	26
Mayo-Almond Face Mask	27
Natural Apple & Sage Face Mask	28
Apricot Face Mask	29
Avocado Face Mask	30
Banana Dry Skin Face Mask	31
Banish Blemishes Face Mask	32
Acne Attack Face Mask	33

Cool Cucumber & Mint Face Mask	34
Oatmeal Face Mask	35
Cornmeal & Egg Face Mask	36
Quick Dry Skin Face Mask	37
Queen's Face Mask	38
3 Fruit Face Mask	39
Green Grape Face Mask	40
Breakfast Face Mask	41
Honey & Oaty Face Mask	42
Tired Skin Face Mask	43
Pretty Papaya & Aloe Face Mask	44
Homemade Face Creams - Intro	45
Jojoba & Aloe Moisturizing Cream	46
Lemon Anti-Wrinkle Cream	47
Mayo Face Cream	48
Simple Olive Oil Face Cream	49
Best Anti-Aging Face Cream	50
Honey Face Cream	51
Vitamin-E Face Cream	52
Citrus Wrinkle Face Cream	53
Ginger Face Cream	54
Aloe Face Cream	55
Green Tea Face Cream	56
Nourishing Face Cream	57
Youth Restoring Face Cream	58
Homemade Eye Creams - Intro	59
Avocado Wrinkle Eye Cream	60
Cocoa Night Eye Cream	61
Almond Eye Tightening Cream	62
Lavender Eye Cream	63
Aloe & Cucumber Eye Gel	64
Conclusion	65
My Other Homemade Beauty Product Books	65

Introduction

In this book, I am giving you **52** of my **Homemade Facial Beauty Products.**

What makes all these recipes fabulous is how quickly you can put these together. Once you have bought a few basic ingredients then you will be able to make lots of products not only for you and your family, but for friends and colleagues too. There's a good chance that you already have many of the ingredients needed to create these products at home.

There is nothing better than going **NATURAL**. What you put on your skin is ever so important. When you make your own face cleansers, face masks and creams, you know **EXACTLY** what is in them and you can alter any recipe to suit yourself. No more unhealthy and dangerous products for you. Natural all the way!

You can create these natural and wholesome beauty products for creating a more youthful glow to your complexion, for helping to relieve feelings of stress and anxiety from your skin and to reverse the signs of aging. You name it, there's a homemade solution for it.

The sky is the limit when it comes to making your own natural beauty products. You are only limited by your own imagination. Anything is possible. Are you ready to feel beautiful?

Lorraine xx

Everyday Products Are Full of Harmful Chemicals

It was five years ago almost to the day that I decided to **STOP** putting harsh chemicals on my skin. This was after I researched the harmful, toxic ingredients that beauty product manufacturers put in our products.

They do this as a money saving exercise mainly and seem to show little if any concern for the end consumer. This made me angry!

The more I looked into the situation, the more I found out about how these toxins silently seep into your system through your skin. I knew that day that I had to be more careful about what I put on my skin. If you have children like me, you will be concerned about what you are putting on them too.

Some of the nasty 'hidden' ingredients in some of my lotions and creams were:

- Synthetic (un-natural) fragrances
- Methlyparaben
- Oxybenzone
- Stearalkonium Chloride
- Diethanolamine
- Propylene Glycol
- Artificial colors

This is just a few that I can remember. When you look these ingredients up, like me, you will be horrified and surprised that these manufacturers get away with it. They not only get away with it, they actually make millions of dollars selling us all potentially harmful and poisonous products.

These manufacturers are so big and powerful that any attempt to try and highlight them for what they are doing generally has no effect.

Rather than accept my toxic fate, I decided to take my own health and beauty matters into my own hands and create my own products. I am proud to say that I haven't bought a shop bought beauty product in the last 5 years and I look and feel better than I have at any other time in my adult life. The treatments have knocked years off how I look and I have lovely, soft supple problem free skin.

Conduct your own research and come to your own conclusions. I would guess though that as soon as you start looking into the harmful chemicals in your products yourself, like me you will abandon these store bought toxic mixtures and start making your own beauty products from the comfort of your home.

Take a look at the simple and easy recipes in this book and let's get started!

Making Your Own Beauty Products

There is nothing more satisfying than making your own natural beauty products. Beautiful face masks, cleansers and creams that you have created yourself out of wholesome natural and organic (where possible) ingredients.

If you implement the use of natural beauty products into your life, you will not only benefit from more radiant and glowing skin, you will also FEEL better because what you put ON your face actually works its way INTO your body.

All the health benefits associated with certain oils, herbs, spices and essential oils will work their magic on you long after you have rubbed them into your skin.

The whole process of cleansing and massaging your face on a daily basis will prove beneficial almost immediately.

Why do you think these fancy spas charge so much for facials? They know the effect their secret (not really secret as I will show you) cleansers, face masks and creams have on the rejuvenation and maintenance of your skin.

Making your own natural face products at home is easy. By the time you have tried a few of these recipes on your face you will be converted and like me, you will find it hard to buy another store bought product again!

How To Be Beautiful - Top Tips

Beauty comes from within. Have you ever heard that? Well it is true to some degree but if you don't feel beautiful on the inside, it is very hard to feel beautiful on the outside.

It will help you to feel beautiful on the inside if your skin looks beautiful on the outside. People will comment just how radiant you look and this will give you more confidence. Then and only then will you feel your best.

How we feel about ourselves as women gets worse every year. Dove (skin care manufacturers) conducted a research study in 2004 with thousands of women from 10 countries around the world. The purpose of the research was to measure women's' 'beauty' levels, in other words, how women felt about themselves and what their levels of esteem was.

The study showed that **only 2%** of women actually considered themselves beautiful. The researchers cited the implications of a global society that narrowly defines beauty by the images that are broadcast across our TV screens in entertainment, advertising and fashion runways as the main problem which has had the most devastating effect on women.

Now I may not be able to do anything to raise your self-esteem, but I can show you some homemade recipes that will help you to get your face into a beautiful state and it is much easier than you think. Having beautiful skin and being the best (beautiful) you can be on the outside can be achieved relatively cheaply too.

You need to **STOP** washing your face with soap to start off (if you are doing this). Because of the nasty chemicals in a lot of the store bought soaps, your skin is stripped of the essential oils it needs to look and feel healthy. Soap is great for washing dishes, getting rid of grease and making those pots and pans shine but it is not good for the face at all. Stop using it now!

My 13 Top Face Care Tips

1. Limit the time you spend in direct sunlight. If you work outside or have to be in the sun a lot, make sure you protect your face by using a sunscreen with a high SPF protection.

2. Always exfoliate your skin at night so that your fresh skin isn't exposed to the sun rays immediately. This will happen if you exfoliate in the morning and then go out into the sun so only do it at night.

3. Drink more water to properly hydrate your skin on a daily basis. The recommended average is eight glasses a day so try to drink at least this much.

4. Drink green smoothies. The essential nutrients in green vegetables and fruit will work wonders for your skin. After only 3 days of drinking healthy green smoothies, I noticed an improvement in my complexion, my skin was less dry and it felt beautifully soft. The more smoothies I drink, the better my skin gets.

5. Cut back on sugar. Sugar is really toxic and it is proven to be the cause of lots of health problems and diseases. It is known to make your skin age faster, it is one of the culprits for bringing on wrinkles and sugar is also associated with giving you breakouts in your skin causing acne.

6. Eat healthily. The best most nutritious food is important if you want to have the best skin that you could possibly have. They say that we are what we eat, if that's the case then make sure you eat the type of foods that are proven to be good for your skin. Plenty of fresh fruits and vegetables.

7. Get enough sleep. I cannot stress enough the importance of getting enough sleep. Limit your sleep and you will suffer the consequences later on. Your body needs time to rest and restore itself and you can only do this with proper and correct sleep.

8. Exercise and keep fit. The importance of regular exercise is widely acknowledged so I don't need to convince you how important it is to get some exercise in. You don't have to sign up at your local gym and can exercise quite easily at home. Take the stairs instead of the lift, park your car or get off the bus a few stops earlier than normal so that you are walking every day, this will improve your fitness and your skin.

9. Keep your face clean. Make sure you wash your face properly in the morning and at night. Use the recipes in this book to keep your face in pristine condition

10. Smile a lot. They say that a frowning face is an aging face. Frowns bring on wrinkles and we don't want that. Smile whenever you can, even when you don't feel like it. This will not only reduce the amount of wrinkles you create, it will also make you feel a whole lot better too.

11. Develop a daily skin care routine. Use facial masks 2 or 3 times a week and exfoliate your skin at least once a week.

12. Look after the skin on your body too. You have to pay attention to the other parts of your body as well. You may be interested in my other books for the best recipes to do that (details at the back of this book)

13. Love yourself. This is probably the most important tip. If you don't love yourself, it will be really hard for someone else to love you and see your true beauty for what it is. Make sure you take time to spend on your own personal grooming, pampering yourself because you really do deserve it.

Basic Set Up & Equipment Needed

You really do not need much at all in terms of equipment to make your own natural face cleansers, masks and creams. The following list really is enough to get started:

- A couple of glass or ceramic bowls (one small, one medium size)
- Spatula or spoon
- Weighing scales
- Small / medium sized pan
- Hand whisk or blender
- Mini chopper / food processor
- Glass jars (make sure to sterilise them before you use them)
- Fruit and vegetables

As I have been making my own products for five years now I also have a good supply of the following which I use in my recipes:

- Coconut Oil
- Shea Butter
- Cocoa Butter
- Olive Oil
- Almond Oil
- Beeswax
- Vitamin E Oil (and capsules)
- A range of essential oils

I use organic when I can and when funds allow but you don't have to. You can get some very high grade oils and butters without an organic certification. I know because I am always trying new ones and some of them are really great.

Whatever grade you decide to use, the quality of your face products will still be better than anything you can buy in the store.

Homemade Facial Cleansers

Cleansing your face is an important beauty ritual. It should be part of your morning and night time beauty routine. As we go about our day to day business, we pick up all kind of dirt and nasty toxins that stick to and pollute our skin. It is important to properly cleanse your face to remove the dirt and grime from your skin. The following recipes are a good collection of homemade facial cleansers you can use to do just that.

Super Simple Cleanser

Ingredients

- 3 tablespoons ground almonds
- 2 tablespoons of almond milk
- 1 teaspoon of lemon juice

Directions

1. Combine all ingredients in a small bowl
2. Apply to your face and rub gently
3. Allow it to stay on your face for 30 seconds
4. Rinse off and dry your face
5. Enjoy your lovely refreshed skin

Moisturizing Face Cleanser

Ingredients

- 1 tablespoons of honey
- 1 tablespoons of oat bran
- 1 teaspoon of cream

Directions

1. Combine all ingredients in a small bowl
2. Apply to your face and rub gently
3. Allow it to stay on your face for 30 seconds
4. Rinse off and dry your face
5. Enjoy your lovely smooth skin

Skin Restoring Fruit Cleanser

Ingredients

- 1 slice of peeled apple
- 2 tablespoons of natural yogurt
- 1 teaspoon olive oil
- 1 teaspoon lemon juice

Directions

1. Combine all ingredients in a food processor or blender
2. Blend until smooth (about 45 seconds)
3. Apply to your face and rub gently
4. Allow it to stay on your face for 30 seconds
5. Rinse off and dry your face
6. Enjoy your lovely refreshed skin

Skin Smoothing Flour Cleanser

Ingredients

- 4 tablespoons flour
- 2 tablespoons of water
- 1 teaspoon sugar

Directions

6. Combine all ingredients in a small bowl
7. Apply to your face and rub gently
8. Allow it to stay on your face for 10 minutes
9. Rinse off and dry your face
10. Enjoy your lovely skin

Tea Tree Cleanser

Ingredients

- 2 tablespoons castor oil
- 3 tablespoons grape seed oil
- 2 tablespoons jojoba oil
- 3 drops tea tree oil

Directions

1. Combine all ingredients in a small bowl
2. Apply to your face
3. Put a hot washcloth over your face
4. Allow your face to steam until the cloth goes cold
5. Rinse off and dry your face
6. Enjoy your lovely softened skin

Lavender Anti-Aging Face Cleanser

Ingredients

- 6 tablespoons grape seed oil
- 10 drops lavender essential oil
- 5 drops geranium essential oil
- 5 drops rose essential oil

Directions

1. Combine all ingredients in a clean dark glass bottle
2. Shake the bottle
3. Apply a small amount to your face and massage to cleanse
4. Rinse off with warm water and a clean wash cloth
5. Enjoy your lovely silky smooth skin

Fresh Orange Cleanser

Ingredients

- 2 tablespoons of brown sugar
- ¾ cup of orange juice

Directions

1. Mix the brown sugar and orange juice together in a bowl
2. Apply to your face and rub gently
3. Allow it to stay on your face for 2 minutes
4. Rinse off and dry your face
5. Enjoy your lovely refreshed skin

Acne Helping Cleanser

Ingredients

- ½ fresh grapefruit
- 1 kiwi fruit
- ¼ cucumber
- ½ lemon

Directions

1. Combine all ingredients in a food processor or blender
2. Blend until smooth (about 45 seconds)
3. Apply to your face and rub gently
4. Allow it to stay on your face for 2 minutes
5. Rinse off and dry your face
6. Enjoy your lovely refreshed skin

Simple Strawberry Cleanser

Ingredients

- 2 strawberries
- 2 tablespoons plain yogurt

Directions

1. Mix the strawberries and yogurt together in a bowl
2. Apply to skin in a circular motion
3. Rub gently
4. Allow it to stay on your face for 2 minutes
5. Rinse off and dry your face
6. Enjoy your lovely well balanced skin

Aloe Gel Face Wash

Ingredients

- ¼ cup aloe vera gel
- 2 tablespoons of almond milk
- 1 teaspoon of rosewater
- 1 tablespoon soapwort extract
- 6 drops lavender essential oil
- 1 Vitamin E oil capsule

Directions

1. Combine all ingredients in a clean container with a tight lid
2. Wet your face and apply the cleanser
3. Rub it into your face for 30 seconds
4. Allow it to stay on your face for an extra 30 seconds
5. Rinse off and dry your face
6. Enjoy your lovely refreshed skin

Baking Soda Cleanser

Ingredients

- 1 tablespoons of honey
- 1 teaspoon of baking soda
- Few drops of water

Directions

1. Combine the honey and baking soda in the palm of your hand
2. Add a few drops of water to form a paste
3. Massage gently into your face
4. Allow it to stay on your face for 60 seconds
5. Rinse off and dry your face
6. Enjoy your lovely refreshed skin

Yogurt Face Cleanser

Ingredients

- 2 tablespoons of plain yogurt
- 1 teaspoon of honey

Directions

1. Combine the two ingredients together
2. Apply to your face and massage in gently
3. Allow it to stay on your face for 60 seconds
4. Rinse off and dry your face
5. Enjoy your calm, clearer skin

Avocado Dry Skin Cleanser

Ingredients

- 1 tablespoons avocado oil
- 1 tablespoon honey
- 2 tablespoons apple cider vinegar

Directions

1. Combine all ingredients in a small bowl
2. Apply to your face and rub gently
3. Allow it to stay on your face for 60 seconds
4. Rinse off and dry your face
5. Enjoy your lovely cleansed skin

Cucumber Face Cleanser

Ingredients

- ½ cup plain yogurt
- ½ cucumber (peeled and deseeded)
- 5 mint leaves

Directions

1. Combine all ingredients in a food processor or blender
2. Blend until smooth (approx. 45 seconds)
3. Apply to your face and massage gently
4. Allow it to stay on your face for 5 minutes
5. Rinse off and dry your face
6. Enjoy your gorgeous clean skin

Lemon & Honey Cleanser

Ingredients

- ½ cup rolled oats
- ½ cup fresh lemon juice
- ¼ cup water
- ½ tablespoon honey

Directions

1. Combine all ingredients in a bowl
2. Apply to your face and massage gently
3. Allow it to stay on your face for 5 minutes
4. Rinse off and dry your face
5. Enjoy your skin

Homemade Face Masks

Homemade face masks are not only a luxurious indulgence, they are also very good for your skin. Whilst cleansing your face twice a day will safely remove the dirt and grime from your face, only by treating your face to a face mask will the impurities be drawn out from beneath your skins top layer. Face masks penetrate deeply and get to the parts that cleansers alone cannot. Treat yourself to these face mask recipes, your face will thank you for it later.

Almond & Honey Face Mask

Ingredients

- 1 tablespoons ground almonds
- 1 teaspoon honey

Directions

1. Combine almonds and honey together
2. Apply to your face and massage gently
3. Allow it to stay on your face for 5 minutes
4. Rinse off and dry your face
5. Enjoy your gorgeous clean skin

Mayo-Almond Face Mask

Ingredients

- ½ cup ground almonds
- 1 teaspoon mayonnaise

Directions

1. Mix almonds and mayonnaise together
2. Apply to your face and massage gently
3. Relax and allow it to stay on your face for 10 minutes
4. Rinse off and dry your face
5. Enjoy your beautiful skin

Natural Apple& Sage Face Mask

Ingredients

- 1 apple (cored and sliced)
- 2 tablespoons honey
- ½ teaspoon sage (fresh or dried)

Directions

1. Combine all ingredients in a food processor or blender
2. Blend until smooth (approx. 45 seconds)
3. Apply to your face and massage gently
4. Allow it to stay on your face for 2 minutes
5. Rinse off and dry your face
6. Enjoy your gorgeous clean skin

Apricot Face Mask

Ingredients

- 2 apricots
- 2 tablespoons plain yogurt
- 5 mint leaves

Directions

1. Combine all ingredients in a food processor or blender
2. Blend until smooth (approx. 45 seconds)
3. Apply to your face and massage gently
4. Relax and allow it to stay on your face for 10 minutes
5. Rinse off and dry your face
6. Enjoy your gorgeous clean skin

Avocado Face Mask

Ingredients

- ½ ripe avocado
- 1 teaspoon vegetable oil

Directions

1. Mix avocado and oil into a paste
2. Apply to your face and massage gently
3. Allow it to stay on your face for 10 minutes
4. Rinse off and dry your face
5. Enjoy your beautiful skin

Banana Dry Skin Face Mask

Ingredients

- 1 ripe banana
- 1 cup oatmeal
- 2 tablespoons milk

Directions

1. Combine all ingredients in a bowl
2. Apply to your face and massage gently
3. Allow it to stay on your face for 10 -15 minutes
4. Rinse off and dry your face
5. Enjoy your gorgeous clean skin

Banish Blemishes Face Mask

Ingredients

- 1 tomato (chopped)
- 1 teaspoon lemon juice
- 1 tablespoon oatmeal

Directions

1. Combine all ingredients in a bowl
2. Mix until smooth
3. Apply to your face and massage gently
4. Allow it to stay on your face for 5 minutes
5. Rinse off and dry your face
6. Enjoy your gorgeous clean skin

Acne Attack Face Mask

Ingredients

- 3 large carrots
- 5 tablespoons yogurt
- 1 teaspoon lemon juice

Directions

1. Combine all ingredients in a food processor or blender
2. Blend until smooth (approx. 45 seconds)
3. Apply to your face and massage gently
4. Allow it to stay on your face for 10 minutes
5. Rinse off and dry your face
6. Enjoy your lovely skin

Cool Cucumber & Mint Face Mask

Ingredients

- ½ cucumber
- 1 tablespoon plain yogurt
- ½ cucumber (peeled and deseeded)
- 3 mint leaves

Directions

1. Combine all ingredients in a food processor or blender
2. Blend until smooth (approx. 45 seconds)
3. Apply to your face and massage gently
4. Allow it to stay on your face for 2 minutes
5. Rinse off and dry your face
6. Enjoy your beautiful silky smooth skin

Oatmeal Face Mask

Ingredients

- ½ cup oatmeal
- ½ cup cornmeal
- 1/3 cup whole milk powder
- ½ cup corn flour
- Few drops of water

Directions

1. Combine all ingredients in a mortar
2. Add a few drops of water and mix until smooth
3. Apply to your face and massage gently
4. Allow it to stay on your face for 3 minutes
5. Rinse off and dry your face
6. Enjoy your gorgeous clean skin

Cornmeal & Egg Face Mask

Ingredients

- 1 tablespoon cornmeal
- 1 egg (whisked)

Directions

1. Cleanse your face with one of the cleansers in this book
2. Massage the cornmeal into your face gently
3. Rinse off and apply whisked egg mixture to your face
4. Allow it to stay on your face for 15 minutes
5. Rinse off
6. Feel your skin, it will be soft and beautiful

Quick Dry Skin Face Mask

Ingredients

- 1 tablespoon oatmeal
- ½ ripe banana (mashed)
- 2 tablespoons plain yogurt

Directions

1. Clean your face with one of the skin cleansers
2. Massage the oatmeal into your face gently
3. Rinse this off
4. Mix the yogurt and banana together into a paste
5. Spread evenly on your face and allow it to stay on your face for 15 minutes
6. Rinse off and dry your face
7. Enjoy your gorgeous radiant skin

Queen's Face Mask

Ingredients

- 1 egg (whisked)
- 1 tablespoon flour
- 1 tablespoon whole milk
- ½ teaspoon olive oil
- ¼ teaspoon sea salt

Directions

1. Mix all ingredients together until you get a paste like consistency
2. Apply to your face evenly and massage gently
3. Allow it to stay on your face for 15 minutes
4. Rinse off and pat dry your face
5. Enjoy your gorgeous clean skin

3 Fruit Face Mask

Ingredients

- ½ ripe banana
- 2 strawberries
- 2 tablespoons crushed pineapple

Directions

1. Combine all ingredients in a bowl and mix together well
2. Apply to your face and massage gently
3. Allow it to stay on your face for 15 minutes
4. Rinse off and pat dry your face
5. Enjoy your gorgeous beautiful skin

Green Grape Face Mask

Ingredients

- 1 cup green grapes
- 1 teaspoon honey

Directions

1. Crush the grapes and honey into a pulp
2. Mix together well
3. Apply to your damp face and massage gently
4. Allow it to stay on your face for 15 minutes
5. Rinse off and dry your face
6. Enjoy your gorgeous clean skin

Breakfast Face Mask

Ingredients

- 1 tablespoon honey
- 1 egg yolk
- 1 tablespoon plain yogurt

Directions

1. Mix all ingredients together very well
2. Apply to your clean damp face and massage gently
3. Relax and allow it to stay on your face for 15 minutes
4. Rinse off and pat dry your face
5. Apply moisturizer of your choice and enjoy your beautiful skin

Honey & Oaty Face Mask

Ingredients

- 1 tablespoon honey
- 1 tablespoon apple cider vinegar
- 1 teaspoon ground almonds

Directions

1. Mix all ingredients together very well
2. Apply to your clean damp face and massage gently
3. Relax and allow it to stay on your face for 15 minutes
4. Rinse off and pat dry your face
5. Apply moisturizer of your choice and enjoy your beautiful skin

Tired Skin Face Mask

Ingredients

- 1 tablespoon ground or powdered spearmint
- 1 tablespoon grape seed oil
- 1 tablespoon honey

Directions

1. Place all ingredients in a blender or food processor
2. Blend until smooth (approximately 45 seconds)
3. Apply to your clean damp face and massage gently
4. Relax and allow it to stay on your face for 15 minutes
5. Rinse off and pat dry your face
6. Apply moisturizer of your choice and enjoy your beautiful skin

Pretty Papaya & Aloe Face Mask

Ingredients

- ¼ ripe papaya
- 4 teaspoons flour
- 1 ½ teaspoons aloe vera gel
- 1 egg yolk
- 1 tablespoon plain yogurt

Directions

6. Mix all ingredients together very well
7. Apply to your clean damp face and massage gently
8. Relax and allow it to stay on your face for 15 minutes
9. Rinse off and pat dry your face
10. Apply moisturizer of your choice and enjoy your beautiful skin

Homemade Face Creams

Face creams are important in locking in all the natural goodness. They help to keep your skin moisturized, hydrated and radiant. If you want a glowing look to your skin, it is important to make sure you lather your face with face creams. Whether you have oily, dry, combination, aging, tired or sensitive skin, there will be a cream here for you. See which one you like best.

Jojoba & Aloe Moisturising Cream

Ingredients

- 25g jojoba oil
- 10 g beeswax
- 10g cocoa butter
- 1 tablespoon vitamin E oil
- 50g aloe vera gel
- 10g glycerine
- 20 drops lavender essential oil

Directions

1. Half fill two small to medium sized pans with water and place on medium heat
2. Put a clear glass bowl on top of each pan so the bowls are immersed in the water
3. Put the jojoba, beeswax, cocoa butter and vitamin E oils in one of the glass bowls
4. Put the aloe vera gel and glycerine in the second bowl
5. Heat both mixtures up until 160 degrees (until well mixed together)
6. Remove both pans from the stove
7. Take the jojoba oil mix and pour it gently into the aloe mixture
8. Allow it to cool for 5-10 minutes
9. Add the lavender essential oil
10. Store in a clean air tight jar

Lemon Anti-Wrinkle Face Cream

Ingredients

- 1 tablespoon beeswax
- 3 tablespoons vegetable oil
- 1 tablespoon witch hazel
- 1 tablespoon lemon juice
- 1/8 teaspoon borax
- 6 drops lemon essential oil

Directions

1. Half fill a small to medium sized pan with water and place on medium heat
2. Put a clear glass bowl on top of the pan so the bowl is immersed in the water
3. Put the beeswax and vegetable oil in the glass bowl
4. Heat the mixture, stirring frequently for about 5 minutes
5. In another bowl gently warm the witch hazel and lemon juice
6. Stir in the borax until fully dissolved
7. Add this witch hazel, lemon juice and borax mixture to the beeswax mixture
8. Whisk together with a fork
9. Once cooled, add the lemon essential oil
10. Store in a clean air tight jar

Mayo Face Cream

Ingredients

- 2 egg yolks
- 1 cup vegetable oil
- 1 teaspoon wheat germ oil
- 1 tablespoon vinegar
- 1/8 teaspoon borax
- 4 drops geranium essential oil

Directions

1. Whisk the egg yolks in a bowl and add half of the oil slowly
2. Mix fast with a whisk for 5 minutes (can be done in blender)
3. Add more of the oil to thicken the mixture
4. Add vinegar, borax and geranium essential oil
5. Store in a clean air tight jar

Simple Olive Oil Face Cream

Ingredients

- ½ teaspoon borax
- 2 teaspoons boiled water
- 4 tablespoons petroleum jelly
- 4 tablespoons olive oil

Directions

1. Dissolve the borax in boiling water
2. In a pan with water, place a clear bowl on top (to create double boiler)
3. Heat the water and melt the petroleum jelly and olive oil in the bowl
4. Add the borax mixture and stir well
5. Remove from heat
6. Whisk rapidly as the mixture cools
7. Store in a clean air tight jar in the refrigerator

Best Anti-Aging Face Cream

Ingredients

- ¼ cup almond oil
- 2 tablespoons coconut oil
- 2 tablespoons beeswax
- ½ teaspoon vitamin E oil
- 1 tablespoon shea butter
- 4 drops geranium essential oil

Directions

1. Put all the ingredients in a glass jar
2. Bring a pan of water to the boil and put the glass jar in it
3. Let all the ingredients melt together stirring occasionally
4. Once completely melted together, pour the mixture into a glass jar

Honey Face Cream

Ingredients

- 3 tablespoons vegetable oil
- 3 tablespoons distilled water
- 2 teaspoons beeswax
- 1 teaspoon honey

Directions

1. Put the beeswax and vegetable oil in a glass jar
2. Bring a pan of water to the boil and put the glass jar in it
3. Let the ingredients melt together stirring occasionally
4. Once completely melted together, gently pour the honey into the oil mixture
5. Whisk continuously and add the distilled water
6. Keep in the refrigerator

Vitamin E Face Cream

Ingredients

- 2 teaspoons plain yogurt
- ½ teaspoon honey
- ½ teaspoon lemon juice
- 3 vitamin E capsules

Directions

1. Stir the yogurt, honey and lemon juice together and mix until combined
2. Open the vitamin E capsules and pour the inner contents into the mixture
3. Place it in a clean glass jar and store it in the refrigerator

Citrus Wrinkle Face Cream

Ingredients

- 1 teaspoon apple juice
- 1 teaspoon lemon juice
- 1 teaspoon lime juice
- 2 tablespoons buttermilk
- 1 teaspoon rosemary leaves
- 3 seedless green grapes
- ¼ pear
- 2 egg whites

Directions

1. In a blender, place all ingredients and blend on medium for 30 seconds
2. Pour the mixture into a glass jar

Ginger Face Cream

Ingredients

- 5cm piece of fresh ginger
- 2 teaspoons light sesame oil
- 2 teaspoons apricot kernel oil
- 2 teaspoons vitamin E oil
- ½ cup cocoa butter

Directions

1. Grate the ginger finely and put it in a glass jar
2. Bring a pan of water to the boil and put the glass jar in it
3. Add the rest of the ingredients
4. Let all the ingredients melt together stirring occasionally
5. Allow to cool and place it in a glass jar

Aloe Face Cream

Ingredients

- 2/3 cup distilled water
- 1/3 cup aloe vera gel
- 2 drops tea tree essential oil
- ¾ cup grape seed oil
- 1/3 cup coconut oil
- ¼ teaspoon lanolin
- 2 tablespoons beeswax
- 2 teaspoons light sesame oil
- 2 teaspoons apricot kernel oil
- 2 teaspoons vitamin E oil
- ½ cup cocoa butter

Directions

1. Combine all ingredients (except the tea tree oil) in a glass jar
2. Bring a pan of water to the boil and put the glass jar in it
3. Let all the ingredients melt together stirring occasionally
4. Allow to cool for 10 minutes and place the mixture in a blender
5. Blend on high for 60 seconds
6. Put it back in the glass jar and store it in the refrigerator

Green Tea Face Cream

Ingredients

- 4 tablespoons hazelnut oil
- 2 tablespoons beeswax
- ½ cup green tea
- 2 tablespoons aloe vera gel
- 4 vitamin E capsules

Directions

1. Put the beeswax and hazelnut oil in a glass jar
2. Bring a pan of water to the boil and put the glass jar in it
3. Add the green tea and the inside of the vitamin E capsules
4. Mix well and allow to cool
5. Place it in the refrigerator in a glass jar

Nourishing Face Cream

Ingredients

- ½ cup coconut oil
- ½ cup shea butter
- ¼ cup almond oil
- 6 drops lavender essential oil

Directions

1. Put the shea butter and coconut oil in a glass jar
2. Bring a pan of water to the boil and put the glass jar in it
3. Allow the mixture to melt together
4. Add the almond oil and mix well
5. Allow to cool in the refrigerator for one hour
6. Remove from jar and put the mixture in a blender
7. Whip it up in the blender for 90 seconds
8. Add lavender essential oil and whip for another 20 seconds
9. Allow to cool and place in a glass jar
10. Keep it in the refrigerator until you are ready to use it

Youth Restoring Face Cream

Ingredients

- 1 tablespoon aloe vera gel
- 1/8 cup distilled water
- 1 tablespoon beeswax
- 1//8 cup lanolin
- 2 tablespoons vegetable oil
- 4 drops geranium essential oil

Directions

1. Combine aloe vera gel and vegetable oil and mix well
2. Bring a pan of water to the boil and get a glass jar
3. Put the beeswax and lanolin in it and heat until melted together
4. Add the distilled water and geranium essential oil
5. Mix well and remove from heat
6. Allow to cool
7. Place it in the refrigerator in a glass jar

Homemade Eye Creams

You have to look after the skin around your eyes as well. Most face and body creams are not suitable for around your eye area because they are too strong for this delicate part of your skin. The following recipes will help to rejuvenate tired skin and help to prevent crow's feet and lines around your eyes. Use one of these recipes a couple of times a week for tip top eyes.

Avocado Wrinkle Eye Cream

Ingredients

- 3 slices of ripe avocado
- 5 drops almond oil

Directions

1. Mash the avocado in a bowl into a fine pulp
2. Add the almond oil and mix well
3. Apply to eye area paying attention to any wrinkles
4. Let the cream stay on for 10–15 minutes
5. Rinse off and enjoy your renewed eyes

Cocoa Night Eye Cream

Ingredients

- 1 tablespoon cocoa butter
- 1 tablespoon lanolin
- 1 teaspoon wheat germ oil
- 1 drop rosemary essential oil

Directions

1. Put the cocoa butter and lanolin in a glass jar
2. In a pan, heat some water and add the glass jar
3. Allow the heat to fuse the cocoa butter and lanolin together
4. Add the wheat germ oil and remove from the heat
5. Add the rosemary essential oil
6. Pour into a clean glass jar
7. When ready, apply around the eyes, working the cream in with your fingers
8. Allow it to work its magic throughout the night

Almond Eye Tightening Cream

Ingredients

- 100 ml boiling water
- 1 sprig rosemary
- 1 teaspoon ground almonds
- 1 egg white

Directions

1. Put the rosemary in a bowl and pour the boiling water over it
2. Set aside and allow to cool (this will infuse the water with the rosemary)
3. When cooled, remove the rosemary and strain the mixture
4. Mix the ground almond, egg white and 2 tablespoons of the rosemary infused water
5. Apply to eye area carefully
6. Let the cream stay on for 10–15 minutes
7. Rinse off and enjoy your renewed eyes

Note: The extra rosemary infused water can be kept in the refrigerator for up to 7 days for when you want to make this eye tightening cream again

Lavender Eye Cream

Ingredients

- ½ cup coconut oil
- 2 vitamin E capsules
- 4 drops lavender essential oil

Directions

1. Put the coconut oil in a bowl and microwave for 10-15 seconds
2. Once in liquid form, pour the inside of the vitamin E capsules in and mix well
3. Add the lavender essential oil
4. Place in a bottle and store it in the refrigerator once cooled

Aloe & Cucumber Eye Gel

Ingredients

- 4 oz aloe vera gel
- ½ large cucumber, washed, deseeded and cut into small chunks

Directions

1. Put the cucumber and aloe vera gel in a blender or food processor
2. Blend until smooth
3. Place in a bottle and store it in the refrigerator
4. Apply this cream around the eyes at night time to help restore tired eyes

Conclusion

Well there you have it, 52 of the best recipes for face cleansers, face masks and face creams. Now go and create some of them yourself and experiment by putting your own unique recipes together as well.

Remember, you are not only putting these natural remedies on your face because they feel nice, you are putting these formulas on your skin because of the enormous amount of moisturizing and health benefits associated with the particular oils and ingredients.

You really owe it to your face to treat it well. Your face is the first thing people see and by adopting a natural skin care routine, you will age better and feel better too. Self-esteem is so closely wrapped up to how we look and feel about ourselves. What better way than to raise your esteem by looking after the first thing people see when they look at you, your beautiful face.

Lorraine Xx

Don't forget to check out my other books in this series, all available on Amazon

- **Homemade Lotion:** 41 All Natural, Simple & Easy To Make Body Lotions, Body Butters & Lotion Bars
- **Homemade Foot Spa**: 48 All Natural Foot Scrubs, Foot Soaks, Foot Creams & Heel Balm Recipes
- **Homemade Body Scrubs** : 52 All Natural, Simple & Easy To Make Body Scrubs, Face Masks, Lip Balms & Body Washes: Amazing DIY Organic & Healing Scrubs To Renew Your Skin & Reverse The Signs Of Aging
- **How To Make Bath Bombs**: *Bath Salts & Bubble Baths: 53 All Natural & Organic Recipes*

Made in United States
Troutdale, OR
01/16/2024